# Sitacise, 30 Seconds Movement/Exercise Chart®

## GREAT FOR THE WHOLE FAMILY, GRANDPARENTS TOO!

Do 30 Seconds every 6 Minutes For Great Health Now!

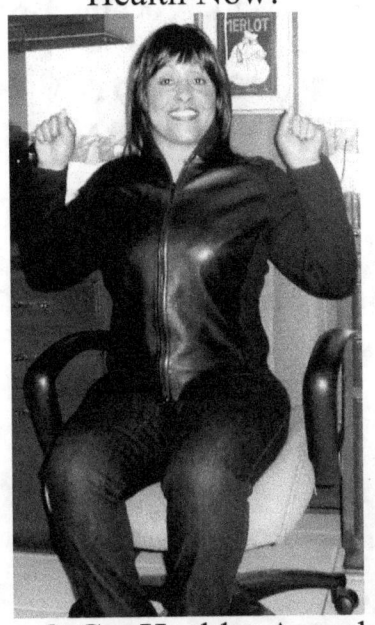

Have Fun & Get Healthy Anywhere You Sit, Is A Place To Get Fit!

At home, at school, at work, in your car, anywhere!

DO 30 SECONDS THEN REST UP TO 6 MINUTES & REPEAT!

Sitacise develops lean muscle that shapes your muscle & burns FAT!

Created by Master Certified Personal Trainers Mark & Kathy Brown

YOU'RE NOT GOING TO GIVE UP YOUR CHAIR SO JUST SIT AND GET FIT THERE!

WE CAN SAVE MILLIONS OF LIVES & BILLIONS OF DOLLARS YEARLY BY DOING SITACISE!

Always consult your care provider before doing this program. Always get a physical before doing these movements!

New revolutionary studies are showing that sitting increases the risks of getting many different diseases and illnesses, even if you exercise 2 HOURS A DAY!

1. Sitting increases the risk of getting "cardiovascular disease" by 54%!

2. Sitting increases the risk of becoming "obese" by over 50%!

3. Sitting almost triples the risks of getting "diabetes"!

4. Sitting causes many back and spine problems, such as leaking discs, herniated discs, nerve damage and severe leg & hip pain!

EVEN IF YOU EXERCISE two hours per day, seven days a week, if you sit for a long period of time those risks are there! It doesn't matter if you are overweight or have a six-pack; smoke or don't smoke, if you sit for long the risks are there.

WHY? Because the fat burning enzyme, lipase is not produced when you sit!

NO FAT BURNING ENZYME, NO FAT BURNING. NO FAT LOST! You increase your chances of being obese by 50%!

# 75% OF ALL AMERICANS ARE SUPPOSED TO BE OBESE BY 2015!

# THE OLD WAYS OF WORKING OUT FOR AN HOUR OR TWO AND KILLING YOURSELF IS NOT WORKING! WHY KEEP DOING ONLY THAT?

# IT'S MUCH TOO HARD & IT WILL NOT GET & KEEP US HEALTHY! EVEN A SIX PACK CAN'T SAVE YOU!

Because of all the modernization that we now have we do not burn the calories that we used to washing dishes, washing clothes, walking to & from school, doing more physical leisure time activities and with our computers that do everything for us from paying the bills to providing us with endless hours of entertainment we sit a lot and don't burn as many calories as we used to doing normal daily activities.

In a new field of study called "Inactivity Physiology" it was found that we don't burn enough "NEAT" or Non Exercise Activity Thermogenisis calories during our day

because of moderation, and that is why Americans as a whole are overweight. We must replace these lost "NEAT" calories or else we will continue to be obese, prone toward diabetes & have increase risks of cardiovascular disease!

But if you do our program and learn our movements you can sit and develop **lean**,

**FAT BURNING MUSCLE DOING 30 SECONDS OF MOVEMENTS EVERY 6 MINUTES! WOW! And you can do it anywhere, in any chair.**

How can 30 seconds every 6 minutes work? It is accumulative, over the course of an hour that is 5 minutes of movement. In a normal 8 hour workday that's 40 minutes of movement. That a lot of "NEAT" replacing calories that are being burned! You can do it every 5 minutes if you want for a bigger calorie burn!

**Americans spend on average 56 hours per week sitting in a seat in a car, at work, in front of a computer or a television. Why not use that sitting time for getting fit time? Learn our Sitacise movements & you can do them anywhere!**

Get Your Sitacise 30 second movement/exercise chart now and start sitting and getting fit today! Why Kill Yourself Working out! Sit & Get Fit & Healthy Now!

NOW YOU DON'T HAVE ANY

EXCUSE FOR NOT BEING HEALTHY &

FIT!

BECAUSE SITACISE IS SO EASY YOU

WILL NOT MAKE ONE! JUST SIT & GET

FIT! EVERYWHERE YOU SIT IS A PLACE

TO GET FIT!

Great for children, Great for parents &
Great for grandparents.
BUY 2, 1 FOR YOU & 1 FOR YOUR
LOVED ONES

Always get a physical before doing these movements!

Next is an example of blood serum samples that were drawn from the same person 15 minutes after he had eaten the same meal. He ate one meal while he was sitting and the blood fats in his system were very thick in the sample on the left because when he sat the enzyme lipase, which places the blood fats in our muscles to be burned as fuel, is not produced.

He ate the same meal while he was standing and the sample is clear of blood fats because the enzyme lipase, was is produced when we stand or move our bodies.

This is why we must move our bodies, even when we sit so that we can become fat burning machines & not fat storing machines.

Something as simple as standing while eating can make such a big difference. Do our Sitacise movements to become a FAT BURNING MACHINE & GET HEALTHY NOW!

Check out our book Sitacise! Just Sit And Get Fit @ www.sitacise.com for more great tips like these.

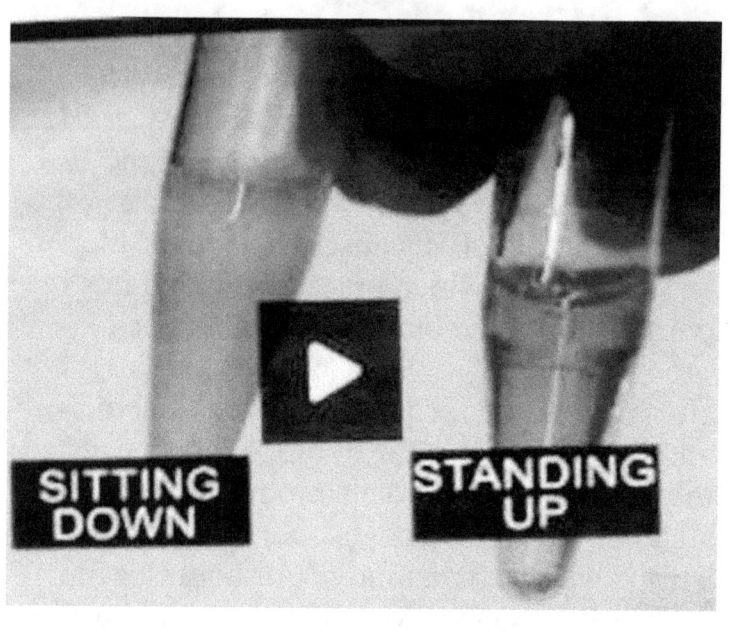

Sitacise 30 Second Exercise/Movement Chart!®

The Chest Press is important to strengthen the two chest muscles: the Pectoralis Major, which is the larger muscle; and the Pectoralis Minor which is the smaller chest muscle. These are sometimes called the pectorals or pecs.

The movement is performed by starting with the feet firmly planted on the floor. Place your back firmly against the seat back; raise your arms to a position that is about chest high & even with your chest. Your fists should be almost even with your chest. Push out from your chest until your arms are almost fully extended but do not lock your elbows. Return to the starting position being aware of keeping your form. You can use resistance such as bottles, weights or bands if you like or flex your muscles during the movement. The movement is illustrated on the following pages.

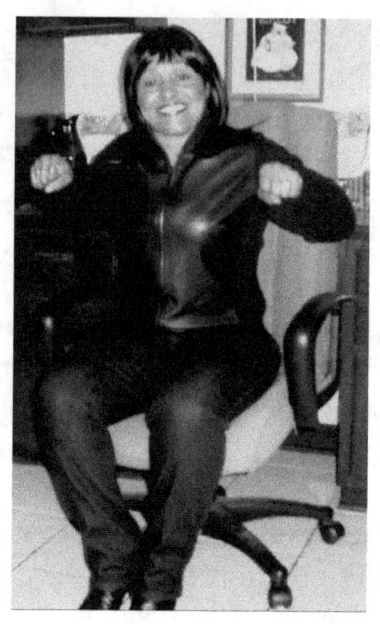

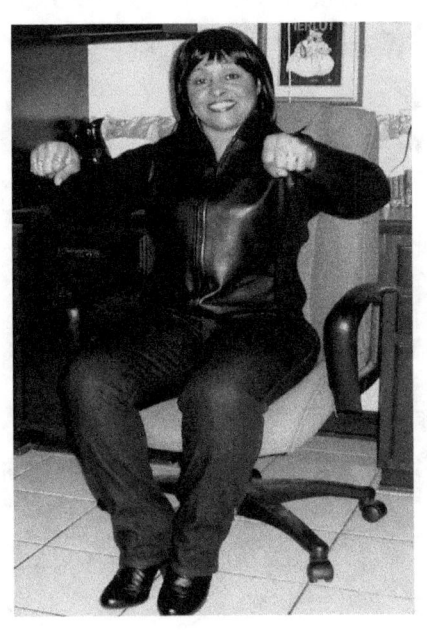

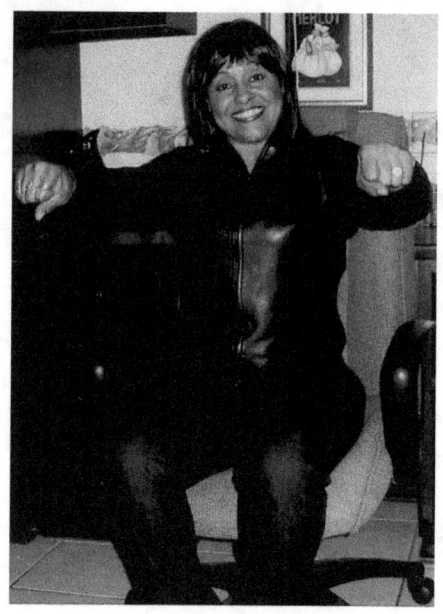

Always get a physical before doing these movements!

Seated Bottle Flies are great for shaping the chest muscles (upper & lower pectorals). Sit with feet firmly on the floor. Raise bottles shoulder width apart & at eye level with elbows facing to the sides. Bring arms together until elbows are facing forward. Slowly return to starting position & repeat until finished or up to 30 seconds. The movement is illustrated on the following pages.

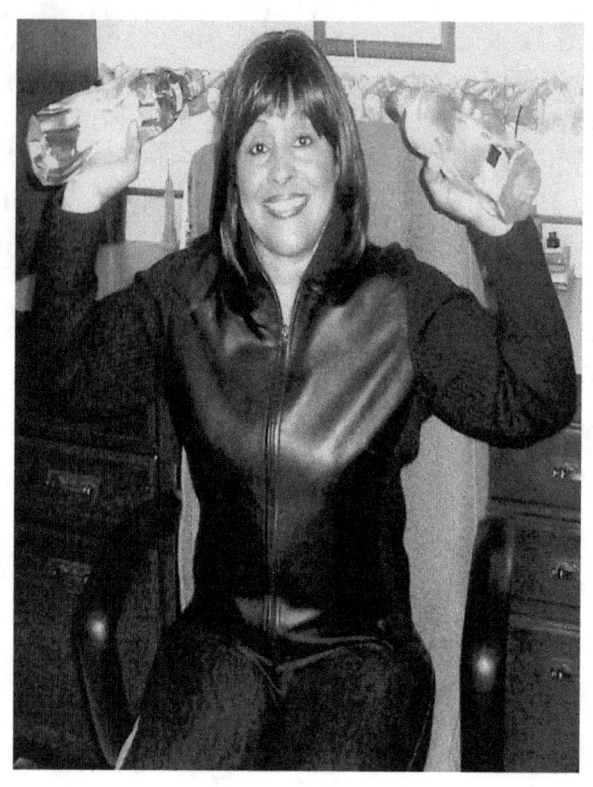

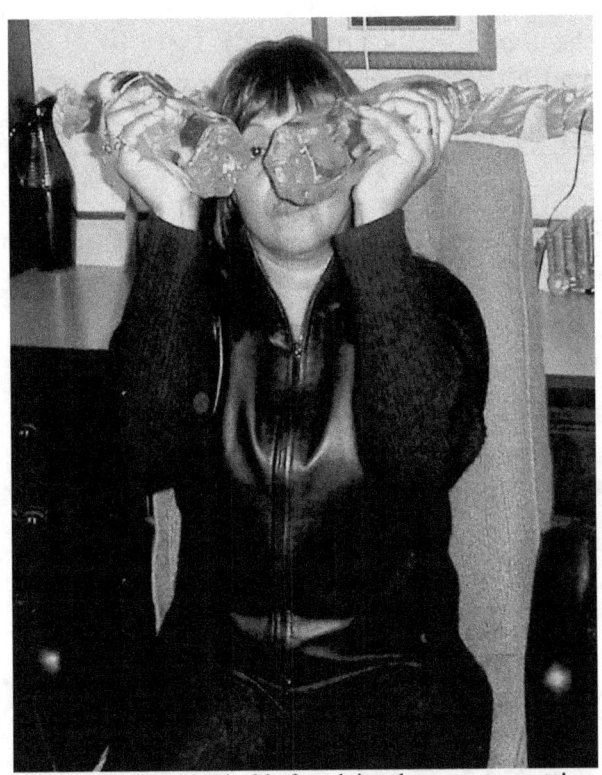

Always get a physical before doing these movements!

The Seated Leg Squat is important to strengthen and firm the thighs, hips, buttocks and hamstrings, as well as strengthening the tendons, ligaments, & bones of the lower body. Begin the movement seating in your chair. Put your hands on the arm of your chair. Make sure the arms of your chair can support you & only use them for balancing, not to support your weight. Rise up by using your legs as the primary source of your power to stand up to a squatting position. Return back to the seated position & then repeat this movement for as long as you can up to 30 seconds. The movement is illustrated on the next page.

The hips, buttocks, thighs & hamstrings are the biggest fat burners in the body!

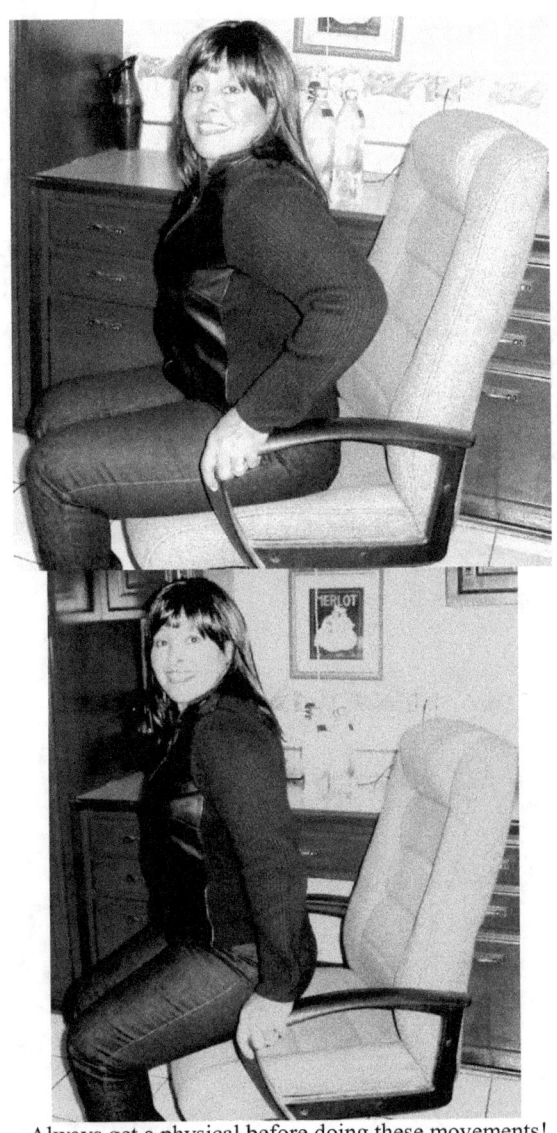

Always get a physical before doing these movements!

The Seated Shoulder Press is important to firm and strengthen the muscles of the shoulders, trapezius & deltoids. Start in the seated position with feet firmly on the floor. Your fists should be almost even with your shoulders. Extend your hands over your head but don't lock out your elbows. Return to the starting position and repeat for as long as you can but no more than 30 seconds. The movement is illustrated on the following pages.

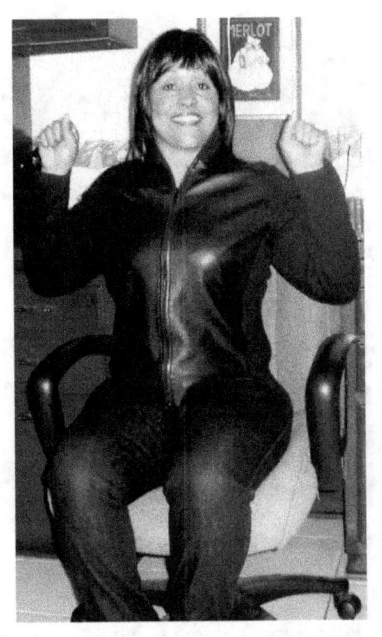

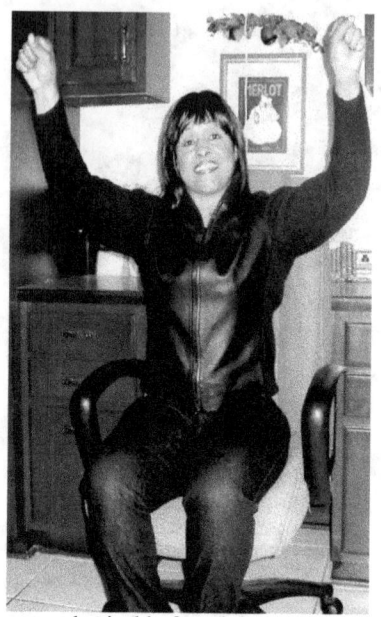

Always get a physical before doing these movements!

The Seated Leg Extension is important to firm & strengthens the quadriceps, the muscles of the front of the thighs. Sit with your feet firmly on the floor. The small of the back should be pressed firmly against the seat back. Extend one leg at a time but do not lock out the knees. Return to starting position & repeat the movement with the other leg & alternate legs as long as you can or up to 30 seconds. The exercise is illustrated on the next page.

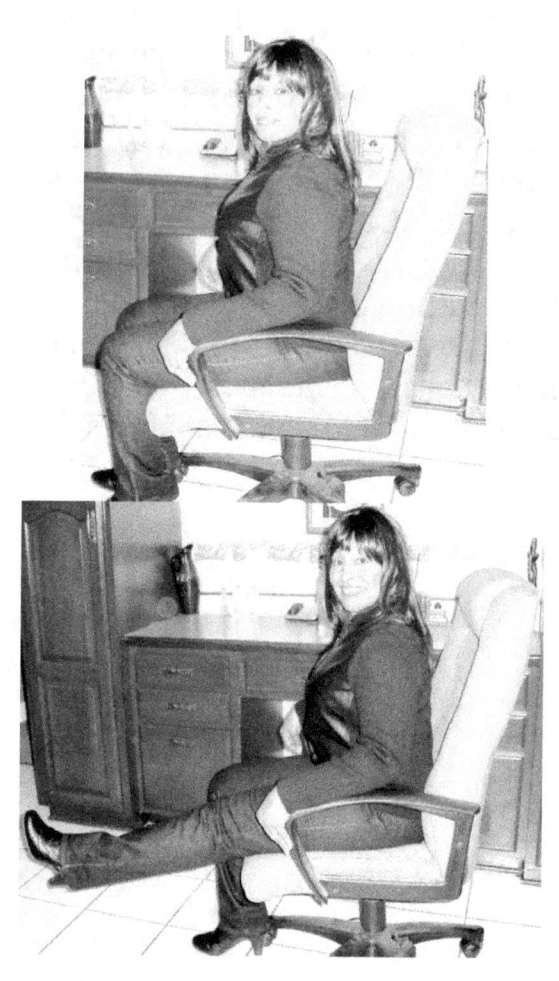

The Standing Alternate Shoulder Press with Water Bottles is important to strengthen & firm the shoulder muscles such as the deltoids & trapezius muscles. Start from a standing position, feet slightly spread. Start with the bottles shoulder high & lift one bottle over your head & as you lower that bottle lift the other bottle over your head, alternating each bottle for as long as you can or for no more than 30 seconds. The Exercise is illustrated below

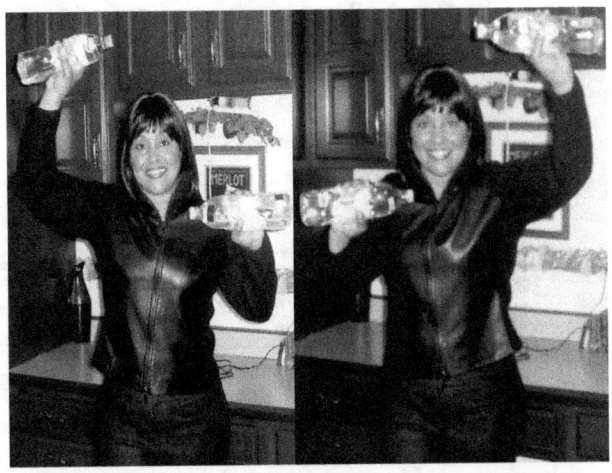

Always get a physical before doing these movements!

Seated Lateral Raises with bottles are important to strengthen & firm up the shoulders, deltoids, and triceps & trapezius muscles. Start with your feet firmly on the floor with your back firmly against the back of the chair. Start with the bottles down at your side and slowly raise them until they are slightly above your shoulders. Slowly lower the bottles until they are back down to your sides. Repeat the movement until you have completed as many as you can or up to 30 seconds of movements. The movement is illustrated on the following page.

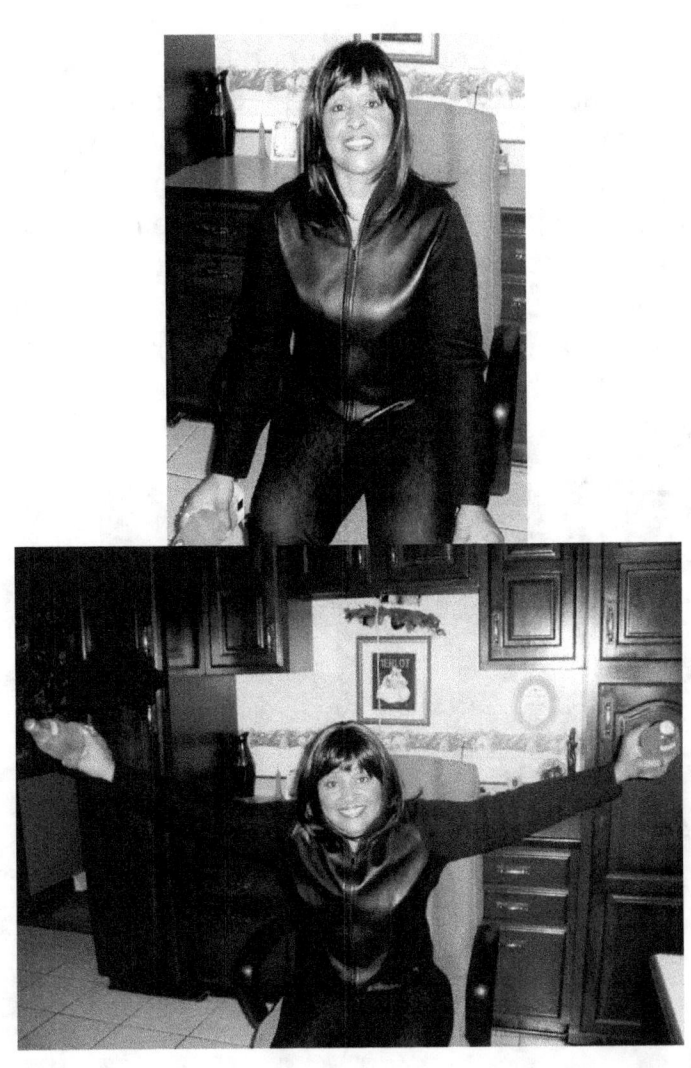

Seated Bottle Presses are good to strengthen the muscles of the shoulder, the deltoids & the Latissimus Dorsi or back muscles. Start with your feet firmly on the floor with your back firmly against the seat. Start with the bottles at shoulder height, raise them over your head but do not lock out your elbows. Return to the start position and repeat the movement for up to 30 seconds. The movement is illustrated here.

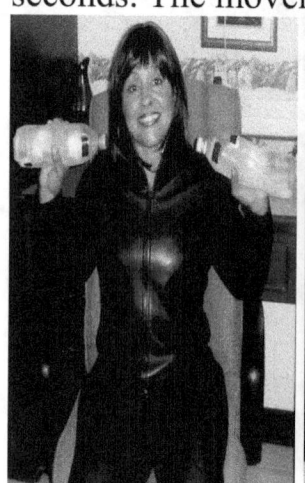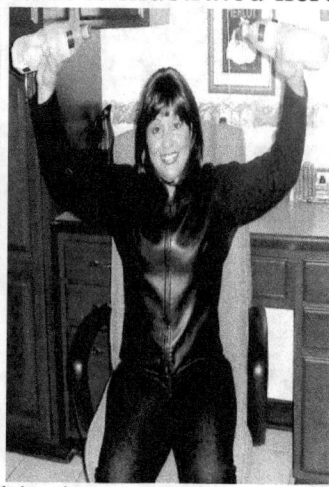

Always get a physical before doing these movements!

Half Squatting is good for firming and developing the thigh muscles, (quadriceps), the gluteus muscles, and (butt) the hip flexors, muscles in the back of the legs, (hamstrings) and the calves. Start by standing beside or in front of your chair, with your feet firmly on the floor. Slightly bend down until you're in a half squatting position, making sure you keep your head up looking straight ahead. You can use your hand for support if you want to. Slowly return to the standing position making sure that you maintain your form. Do as many as you are comfortable with up to 30 seconds. The movement is illustrated on the next page.

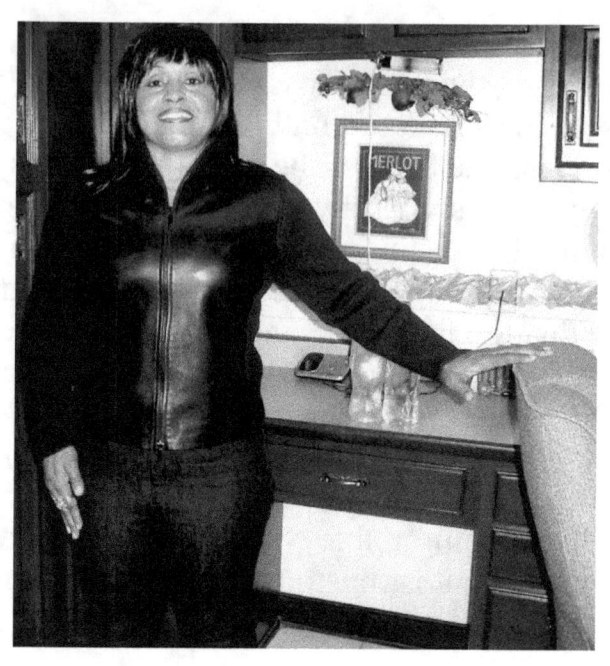

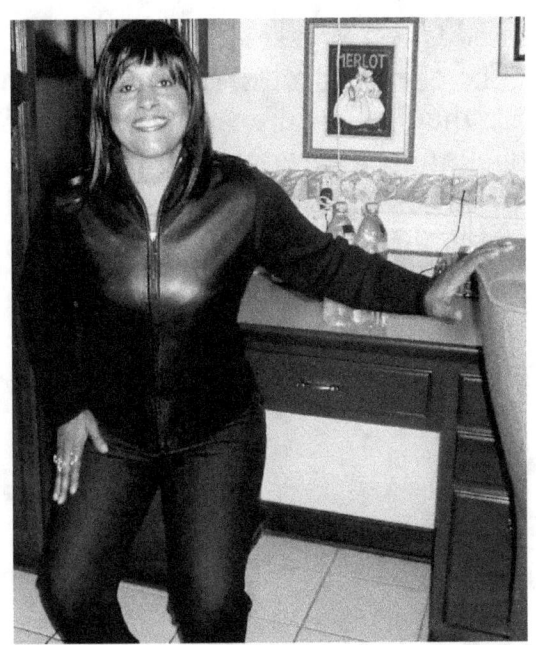

Always get a physical before doing these movements!

The Seated Chest Press with bottles is great for firming the chest muscles, (pectorals) the forearms, the back of the arms, (triceps) & the upper back muscles, (lats). Start with the feet firmly on the floor. Hold bottles chest high & push straight out, do not lock out the elbows. Slowly return to the starting position and repeat as often as desired up to 30 seconds. The exercise is illustrated on the next pages.

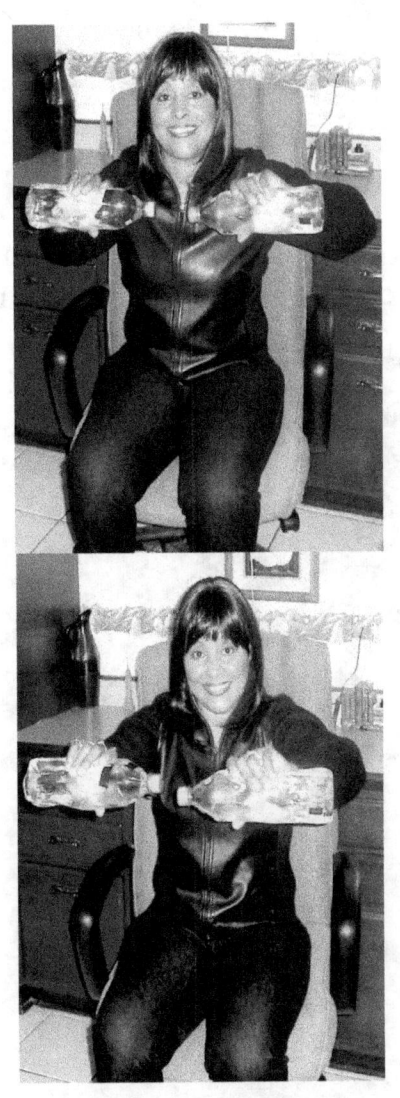

The Seated Calves Raises are great for firming & building the calves muscles of the leg. Start with the feet firmly on the floor. Raise the heel of your foot off the floor while leaving the toes firmly on the floor. Slowly return to the starting position & repeat until finished or 30 seconds are up. The movement is illustrated below.

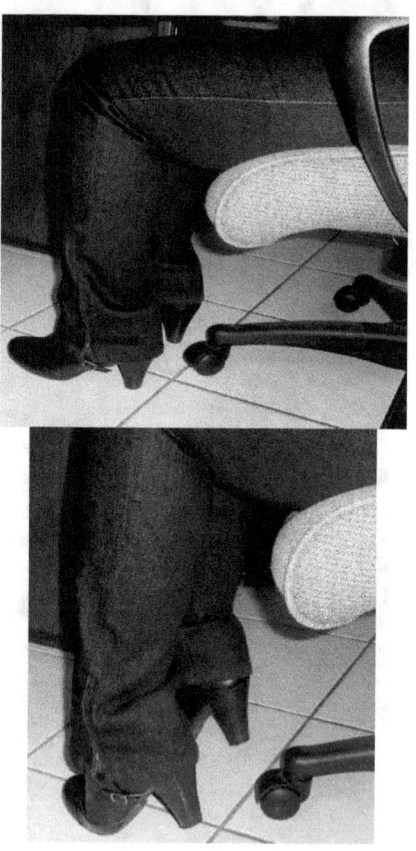

The Standing Side Leg Raise is great for shaping & firming the outside of the leg (abductors) & the gluteus (butt) muscles. Stand with your feet firmly on the floor, knees & feet pointing forward. Use a chair to hold on to for support and tighten your abs & slowly raise your leg out to the side keeping your leg firm. Return to the starting position & repeat until finished or up to 30 seconds. Switch & do the other leg. The movement is illustrated on the following page.

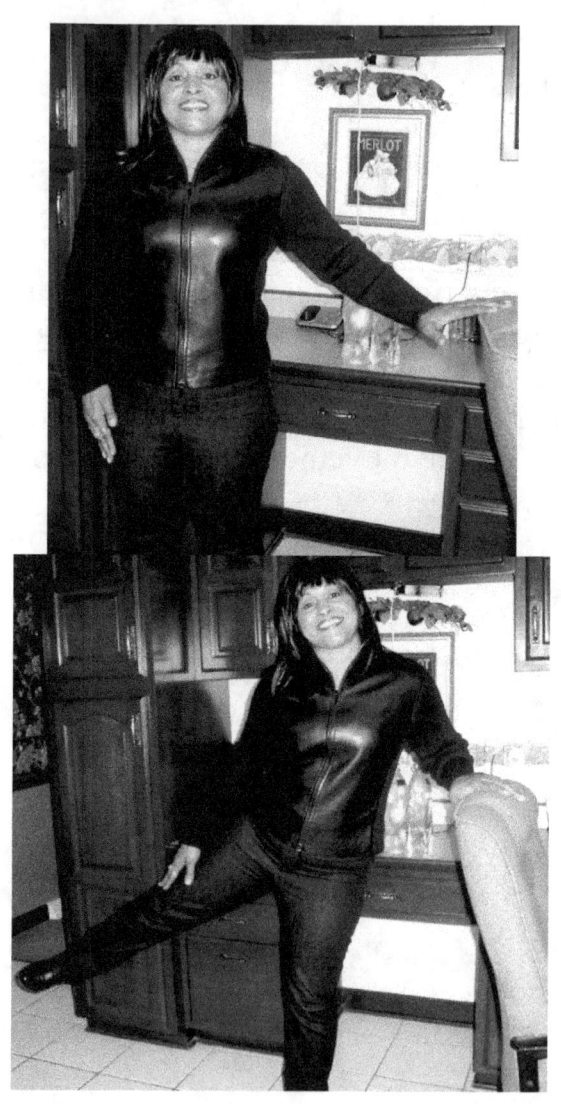

The Standing Front Leg Raise is great for shaping & strengthens the front of the legs (quadriceps). Start with both feet firmly on the floor. Raise your foot & leg out & up to about knee high keeping your leg firm. Return to starting position & repeat until finished or up to 30 seconds. Change legs & repeat with it until finished. The movement is illustrated below

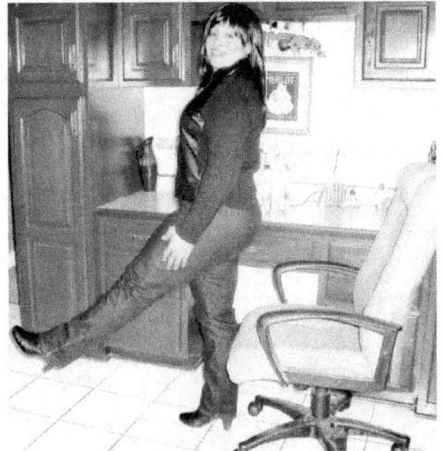

Always get a physical before doing these movements!

The Seated Shoulder Bottle Press is great for strengthening & shaping the shoulders, deltoids, triceps & clavicle. Start with feet firmly on the floor. With your back firmly against the seat back hold each bottle at shoulder height with the elbows facing downward. Raise the bottles overhead until the elbows are almost extended but do not lock out the elbows. Return to the starting position & repeat until you have finished or up to 30 seconds. The movement is illustrated below.

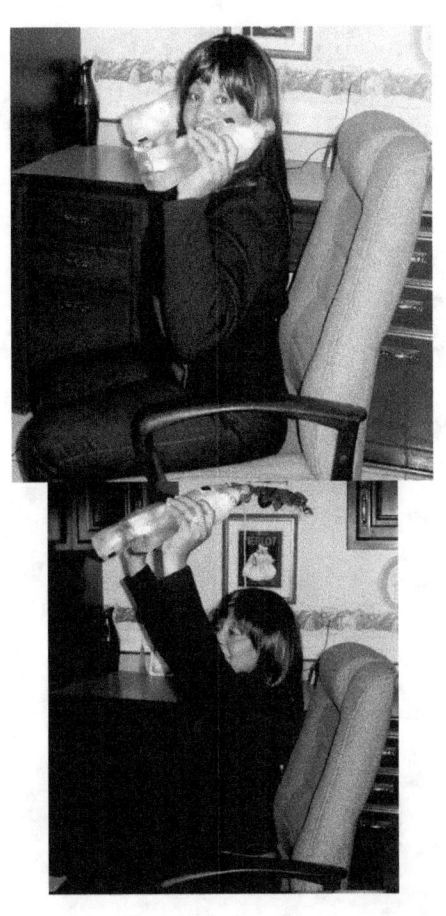

Upright Rowing is great for strengthening & firming the muscles of the shoulders & the biceps. Stand with the feet firmly on the floor, shoulder width apart, the bottles are waist high. Raise the bottles slowly until they are even with your chest your elbows should be pointing outward. Slowly return to the starting position & repeat until finished or up to 30 seconds. The movement is illustrated on the following page.

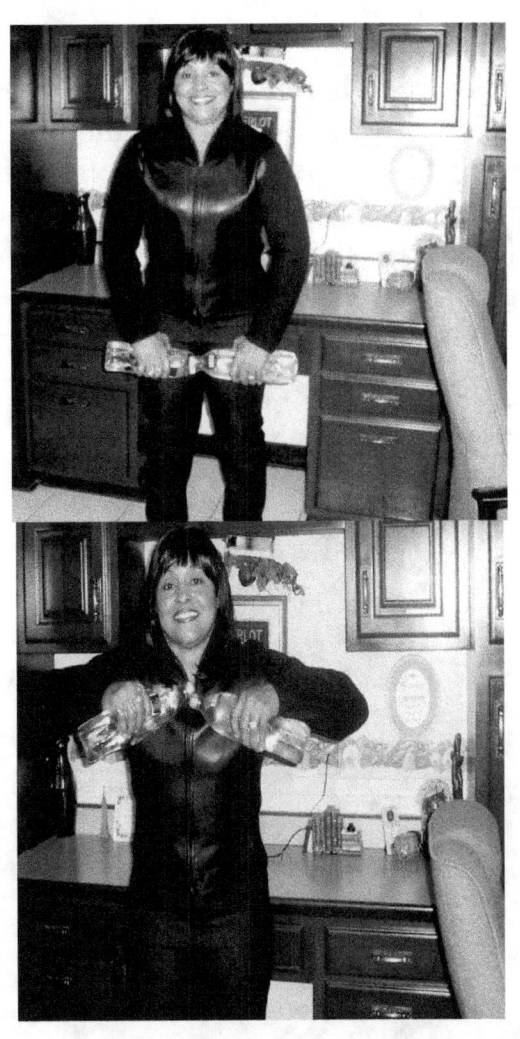

The Seated Curl with bottles is great for firming & strengthening the biceps, forearm and wrist of the arms. Start with the feet firmly on the floor. Hold the bottles to your sides near the top of your thighs. Slowly raise the bottles up until they are shoulder high. Return to the starting position & repeat for up to 30 seconds. The movement is illustrated below.

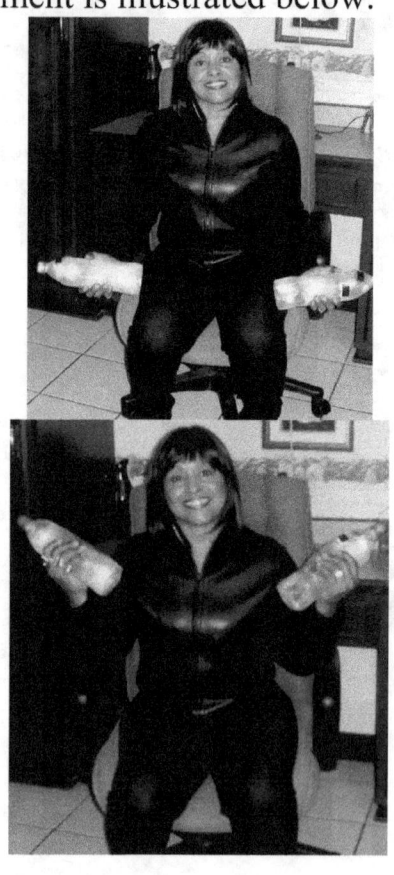

The Desk Push Press is great for strengthening & firming the chest muscles & the back of the arms. Start with your feet firmly on the floor, sitting with the buttocks in the middle of the seat & the upper body leaning forward. Put hands firmly on the desk & push your upper body back until your arms are extended, but don't lock out your elbows. Return to the starting position & repeat until finished or up to 30 seconds. The movement is illustrated on the next page.

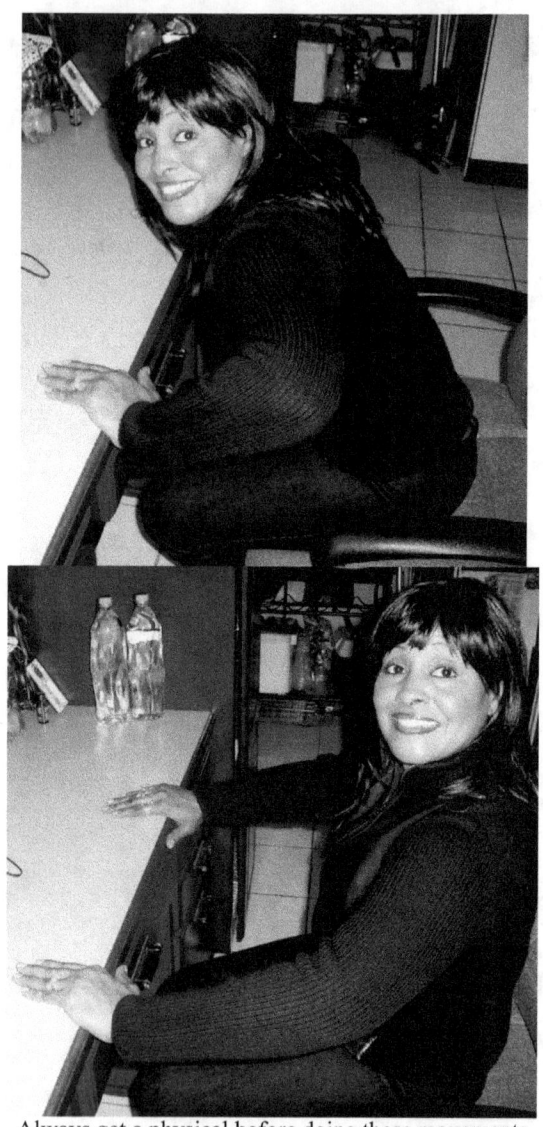

Always get a physical before doing these movements

The Standing Bottle Curl is a great movement to strengthen & firm your arms (biceps) and forearms. Start from the standing position with the bottle just below your waist. Raise the bottle on an angle toward the middle of your chest. Return to the starting position & repeat until finished or up to 30 seconds. Switch arms and repeat until finished or up to 30 seconds. The movement is illustrated on the next page.

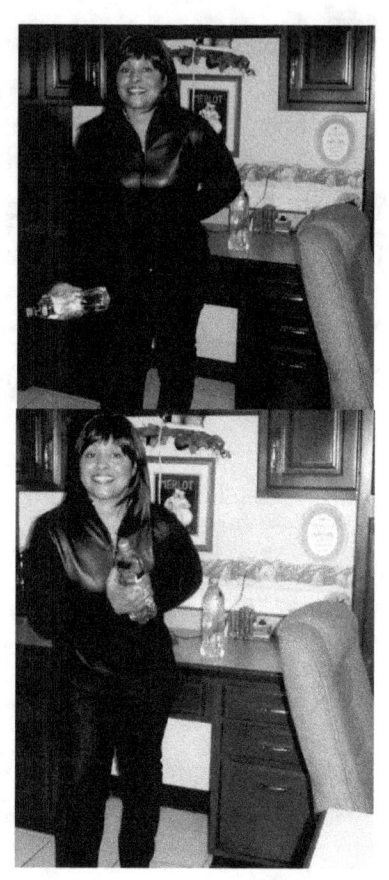

Standing Bottle Flies are great to firm & strengthen the chest muscles (pectorals). From a standing position start with the bottles chest high in each arm in front of the chest. Spread the arms until they are even with the shoulders. Return to the starting position & repeat until finished or up to 30 seconds. The movement is illustrated on the next page.

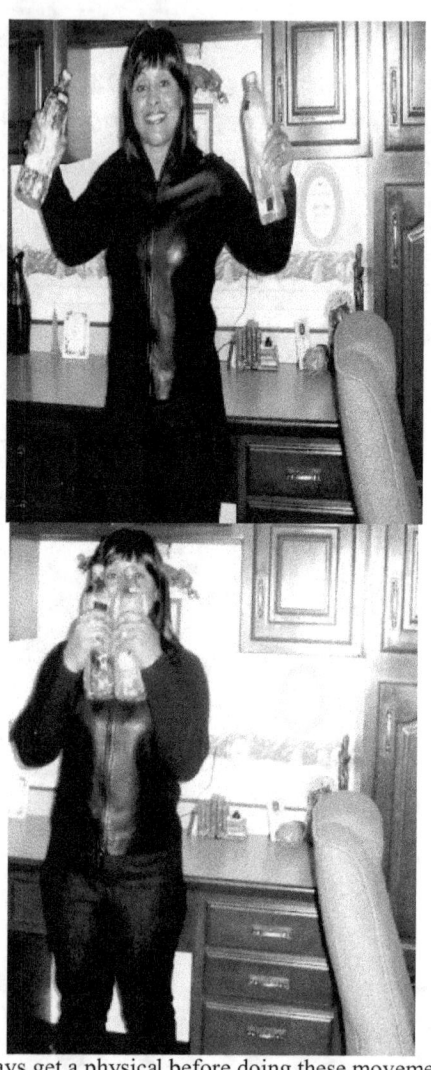

Always get a physical before doing these movements!

The Seated Curl is great to firm & strengthen the biceps & forearms. Start with hands even with the thighs & raise the arms slowly & with tension until your fists are even with your shoulders. Return to starting position & repeat until finished or up to 30 seconds. The movement is illustrated on the next page.

Always get a physical before doing these movements!

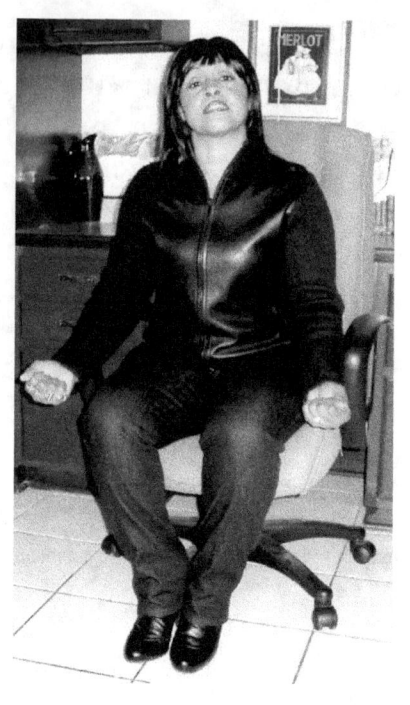

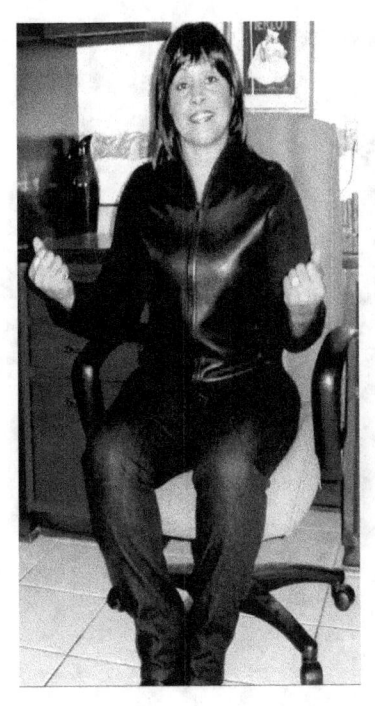

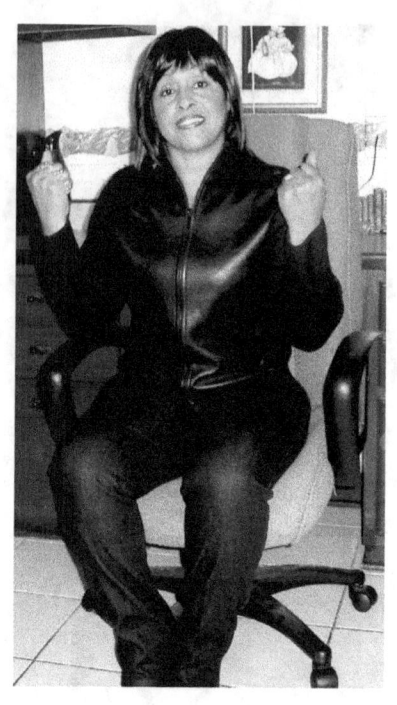

The Seated Fly is great for strengthening &
firming the chest. Start with the fists together
& chest high. Spread your arms until they are
even with the shoulders return to the starting
position & repeat until finished or up to 30
seconds. The movement is illustrated on the
next page.

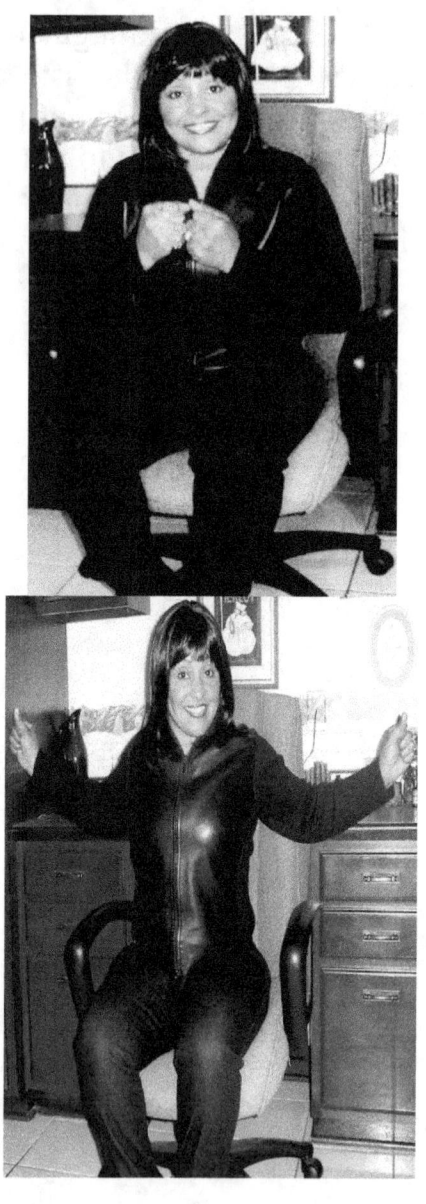

Seated Front Raises with water bottles are great for strengthening & firming the shoulders & chest muscles. Start with the bottles on the lap & raise them overhead. Return to the starting position & repeat until finished or up to 30 seconds. The movement is illustrated on the next page.

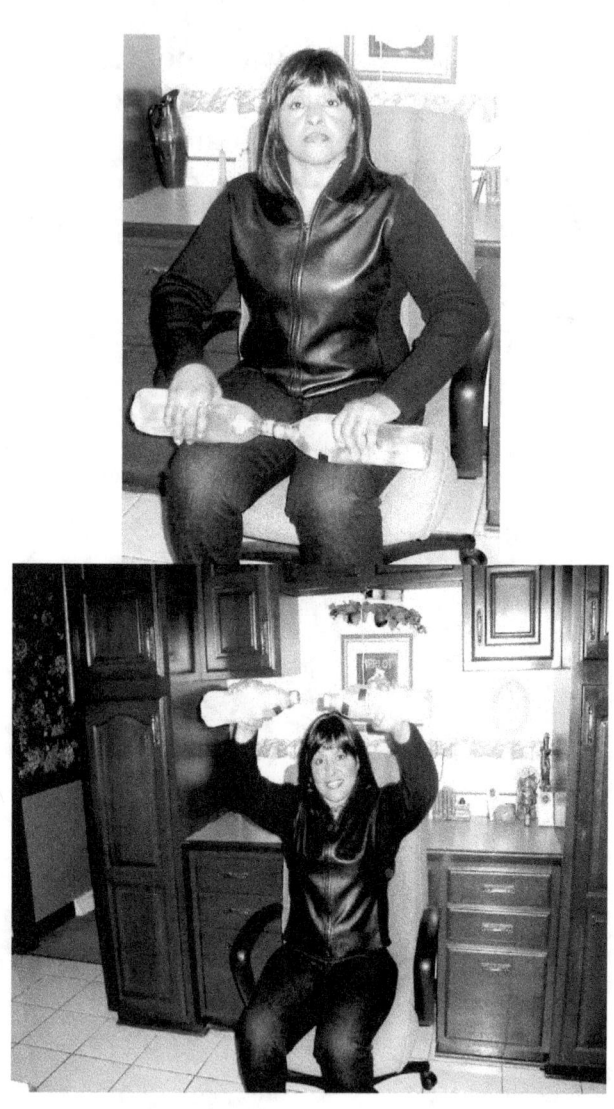

Always get a physical before doing these movements!

If you would like to do more that 30 seconds or if you would like to increase the frequency of the movements/exercises to 3,4,5 minutes for even more calorie burn that is okay, but make certain that you get a physical before you start this movement/exercise program to ensure that you are fit enough to do it.

Our mission is to help as many people as we can to become healthy and if you follow this program you will find that you can do it while maintaining your normal daily activities.

We are only helping you to burn those calories that you use to burn doing the normal daily activities that we used to do. We think that if you can work it in to your normal schedule without any disruption you will be more likely to do it. We just need to keep it simple as possible & that will eliminate a lot of reasons for not doing the program.

Along that line we also have a very simple eating plan that is easily followed.

A healthy eating plan:

- Emphasizes fruits, vegetables, whole grains, and fat-free or low-fat milk and milk products

- Includes lean meats, poultry, fish, beans, eggs, and nuts

- Is low in saturated fats, *trans* fat, cholesterol, salt (sodium), and added sugars

- Controls portion sizes

# Calories

To lose weight, most people need to reduce the number of calories they get from food and beverages (energy IN) and increase their physical activity (energy OUT).

For a weight loss of 1–2 pounds per week, daily intake should be reduced by 500 to 1,000 calories. In general:

- Eating plans that contain 1,000–1,200 calories each day will help most women lose weight safely.

- Eating plans that contain 1,200–1,600 calories each day are suitable for men and also may be appropriate for women who weigh 165 pounds or more or who exercise regularly.

# 1,200 Calories per day

| Breakfast | Energy (Kcal) | Fat (GM) | %Fat |
|---|---|---|---|
| Whole-wheat bread, 1 med. slice | 70 | 1.2 | 15 |
| Jelly, regular, 2 tsp | 30 | 0 | 0 |
| Cereal, shredded wheat, ½ C | 104 | 1 | 4 |
| Milk, 1%, 1 C | 102 | 3 | 23 |
| Orange juice, ¾ C | 78 | 0 | 0 |
| Coffee, regular, 1 C | 5 | 0 | 0 |
| **Breakfast Total** | **389** | **5.2** | **10** |

| Lunch | Energy (Kcal) | Fat (GM) | %Fat |
|---|---|---|---|
| Roast beef sandwich | | | |
| Whole-wheat bread, 2 med. slices | 139 | 2.4 | 15 |
| Lean roast beef, unseasoned, 2 oz | 60 | 1.5 | 23 |
| Lettuce, 1 leaf | 1 | 0 | 0 |
| Tomato, 3 med. slices | 10 | 0 | 0 |
| Mayonnaise, low-calorie, 1 tsp | 15 | 1.7 | 96 |
| Apple, 1 med. | 80 | 0 | 0 |
| Water, 1 C | 0 | 0 | 0 |

| | Lunch Total | 305 | 56 | 16 |
|---|---|---|---|---|

| Dinner | Energy (Kcal) | Fat (GM) | %Fat |
|---|---|---|---|
| Salmon, 2 oz edible | 103 | 5 | 40 |
| Vegetable oil, 1½ tsp | 60 | 7 | 100 |
| Baked potato, ¾ med. | 100 | 0 | 0 |
| Margarine, 1 tsp | 34 | 4 | 100 |
| Green beans, seasoned with margarine, ½ C | 52 | 2 | 4 |
| Carrots, seasoned | 35 | 2 | 0 |
| White dinner roll, 1 small | 70 | 2 | 26 |
| Iced tea, unsweetened, 1 C | 0 | 0 | 0 |
| Water, 2 C | 0 | 0 | 0 |
| **Dinner Total** | **454** | **20** | **39** |

| Snack | Energy (Kcal) | Fat (GM) | %Fat |
|---|---|---|---|
| Popcorn, 2½ C | 69 | 0 | 0 |
| Margarine, ¾ tsp | 30 | 3 | 100 |

| **Grand Total** | **1,247** | **34–36** | **24–26** |
|---|---|---|---|

| | | | |
|---|---|---|---|
| Calories: 1,247 | | SFA, % kcals: 7 | |
| Total Carb, % kcals: | 58 | Cholesterol, mg: 96 | |
| Total Fat, % kcals: | 26 | Protein, % kcals: 19 | |
| Sodium,* mg: 1,043 | | | |

# 1,600 Calories per day

| Breakfast | Energy (Kcal) | Fat (GM) | %Fat |
|---|---|---|---|
| Whole-wheat bread, 1 med. slice | 70 | 1.2 | 15 |
| Jelly, regular, 2 tsp | 30 | 0 | 0 |
| Cereal, shredded wheat, ½ C | 104 | 1 | 4 |
| Milk, 1%, 1 C | 102 | 3 | 23 |
| Orange juice, ¾ C | 78 | 0 | 0 |
| Coffee, regular, 1 C | 5 | 0 | 0 |
| Milk, 1%, 1 oz | 13 | .03 | 23 |
| **Breakfast Total** | **505** | **6.5** | **10** |

| Lunch | Energy (Kcal) | Fat (GM) | %Fat |
|---|---|---|---|
| Roast beef sandwich | | | |
| Whole-wheat bread, 2 med. slices | 139 | 2.4 | 15 |
| Lean roast beef, unseasoned, 2 oz | 60 | 1.5 | 23 |
| American cheese, low-fat and low-sodium, 1 slice (¾ oz) | 46 | 1.8 | 36 |
| Lettuce, 1 leaf | 1 | 0 | 0 |
| Tomato, 3 med. slices | 10 | 0 | 0 |

| Mayonnaise, low-calorie, 2 tsp | 30 | 3.3 | 99 |
|---|---|---|---|
| Apple, 1 med. | 80 | 0 | 0 |
| Water, 1 C | 0 | 0 | 0 |
| **Lunch Total** | **366** | **9** | **22** |

| Dinner | Energy (Kcal) | Fat (GM) | %Fat |
|---|---|---|---|
| Salmon, 3 oz edible | 155 | 7 | 40 |
| Vegetable oil, 1½ tsp | 60 | 7 | 100 |
| Baked potato, ¾ med. | 100 | 0 | 0 |
| Margarine, 1 tsp | 34 | 4 | 100 |
| Green beans, seasoned with margarine, ½ C | 52 | 2 | 4 |
| Carrots, seasoned with margarine, ½ C | 52 | 2 | 4 |
| White dinner roll, 1 med. | 80 | 3 | 33 |
| Ice milk, ½ C | 92 | 3 | 28 |
| Iced tea, unsweetened, 1 C | 0 | 0 | 0 |
| Water, 2 C | 0 | 0 | 0 |
| **Dinner Total** | **625** | **28** | **38** |

| Snack | Energy (Kcal) | Fat (GM) | %Fat |
|---|---|---|---|
| Popcorn, 2½ C | 69 | 0 | 0 |
| Margarine, 1½ tsp | 28 | 6.5 | 100 |
| **Grand Total** | **1,613** | **50** | **28** |

| | |
|---|---|
| Calories: 1,613 | SFA, % kcals: |
| Total Carb, % kcals: 55 | Cholesterol, mg: |
| Total Fat, % kcals: 29 | Protein, % kcals: |
| Sodium,* mg: 1,341 | |

These meal plans should help you to reach your goals to become fit & healthy! You may add to or modify these plans as suits your fitness goals and by all means consult your health care professional for suggestions.

Please remember our illustration of what happens to the production of lipase and the effect it had on fat absorption when one is sitting down and eating and when one is standing up and eating. Simple little tips such as that can save you countless hours of trying to get off the fat that didn't get absorbed.

Because Sitacise is the only program designed specifically to replace those daily "NEAT" Non Exercise Activity Thermogenesis calories that we are not getting, it will eliminate the risks of many illnesses as well as get us fit.

Below is a list of activities; some are exercises & some regular daily activities. You will be amazed at how many calories you can burn just playing cards, driving, or doing housework. Squatting burns 100 calories every ten minutes.

Activity Calories burned: Sleeping 34 Reading 38 Talking on phone 38 Writing 38 Sitting / resting 38 Standing 60 Sex – foreplay 63 Card playing 58 Playing board games 58 Studying 67 Driving 77 Touring/Traveling 77 Packing Suitcase 77 Washing dishes 82 Ironing 82 Shopping 86 Billiards 91 Brush teeth 91 Football - playing catch 91 Croquet 91 Horseback riding – walking 91 Tailoring, Cutting 96 Push stroller with child 96 Putting away Groceries 96 Hairstyling 96 Cooking 96 Walking 2 mph 101 Hatha yoga 101 Playing Piano 101 Housework 106 Frisbee playing 110 Surfing 110 Bowling 110 Dancing - ballroom slow 110 Fishing 110 Loading/Unloading a car 115 Playing guitar 115 Archery 125 Golf – cart 125 Snowmobiling 125 Volleyball – recreation 125 Weight lifting – general 125 Lifting weights – general 125 Pilates

Beginner 134 Carrying an Infant 134 Hang
Gliding 134 Carpentry/Workshop 134 Weaving
cloth 134 Paddleboat 144 Walk / run play with
kids 144 Raking lawn 144 Coaching - team sports
144 Table tennis 144 Water Aerobics 144 Bicycling
– leisure 144 Stretching 144 Showering 154 Sex –
intercourse 154 Elder care, Disabled adult 154
Tennis – doubles 154 Walking 3 mph 158 Mowing
– push 158 Volleyball – competitive 158 Washing
car 163 Calisthenics / exercise - moderate163
Situps / crunches - moderate163 Basketball -shooting
baskets163 Jumping jacks - moderate163
Badminton 163 Mopping 163 Canoeing 2 mph
163 Farming/Feeding livestock 173 Hunting 182
Cricket 182 Painting House 182 Skating –
moderate 182 Softball or baseball 182
Skateboarding 182 Kayaking 182 Pushups –
moderate 182 Ashtanga yoga 187 Pilates
Intermediate 187 Power yoga 187 Walking 4 mph
187 Hopscotch/Dodge ball 192 Using Crutches
192 Snorkeling192 Cleaning Gutters 192 Garden
197 Dancing - fast ballroom 202
Construction/Remodeling 211 Dancing - aerobic,
ballet, modern 216 Boxing - punching bag 216
Horse grooming 216 Fencing 216 Hiking 216
Skiing – water 216 Chop Wood 221 Tennis –
singles 221 Aerobics - low impact 221 Golf - carry
clubs 221 Swimming – moderate 221 Lifting
weights – vigorous 221 Shovel Snow 221 Weight
lifting – vigorous 221 Pilates Advanced 230
Horseback riding – trotting 235 Rearranging
Furniture 240 Sledding, tobogganing 250 Step
aerobics - low impact 254 Racquetball casual 254

Stair Step Machine 254 Basketball – officiating 254 Bikram / hot yoga 254 Rowing machine – moderate 254 Aerobics - high impact 254 Soccer casual 254 Jogging 254 Stationary bicycle / spinning – moderate 254 Backpacking 269 Repelling 293 Situps / crunches – vigorous 293 Horseback riding – galloping 293 Hockey 293 Walking - up stairs 293 Calisthenics / exercise – vigorous 293 Jumping jacks – vigorous 293 Basketball 1/2 court 298 Bicycling / biking – mountain 307 Pushups – vigorous 307 Running 5 mph 307 Frisbee, Ultimate 307 Lacrosse 307 Rowing machine – vigorous 317 Skiing – downhill 317 Football – touch 317 Bicycling / cycling 12-14 mph 317 Vinyasa yoga 317 Skating – vigorous 331 Canoeing 4 mph 336 Football - full contact 350 Ski machine 350 Swimming – vigorous 355 Racquetball competitive 365 Rope jumping 365 Soccer competitive 365 Judo - martial arts 365 Running 6 mph 365 Bicycling / cycling 14-16 mph 384 Step aerobics - high impact 384 Rugby 384 Basketball full court 398 Squatting 300 Rock climbing 398 Skiing - cross country 413 Elliptical trainer 413 Stationary bicycle / spinning – vigorous 413 Running 7 mph 418 Boxing - in ring 437 Handball 437 Running 8 mph 490 Running 10 mph 653 Running 12 mph 811 This is for 30 minutes per activity.

As you can see we can burn lots of calories doing "NEAT" activities without killing ourselves or doing any additional workouts or exercises. When we start to understand that it is not necessary to kill ourselves to be healthy & fit as a nation but that we must do "NEAT" activities and our "Sitacise movements" we will cure the obesity epidemic, reduce the incidence of diabetes & cardio vascular disease & we will also eliminate many back ailments. These diseases cost us over 600 billion dollars per year.

We now have 12 & 13 year old children that are suffering from obesity, diabetes, spinal deformities and many other diseases that were once only seen in adults. Much of these diseases are caused by extended periods of sitting but once they start doing our "Sitacise movements consistently, these conditions will be eliminated. We must do this for the children, our future & ourselves.

Experts are predicting that 75% of all Americans will obese by 2015! Almost 75% of all Americans do not work out! Why don't they do it? Most say they don't have time to workout!

Many say the workouts are just to hard or they are not able to do them because of previous injuries or other physical problems.

Now there is a program that they can do during the normal course of their day, that will help reduce the risks of their being obese by 50%, will reduce the risks of getting diabetes 3 fold, & reduce the risks of getting cardiovascular disease by 54%. This program will also eliminate many back problems, save millions of lives and billions of dollars in health care costs yearly.

Sitacise is the movement/exercise program of the future available today; get yours & start getting healthy & fit now! Thank you for buying our movement/ exercise chart & check out our other products on www.sitacise.com like the Sitacise! Just Sit & Get Fit book & our fitness DVD's. They will change your life & your love ones lives too.

Thank you for buying our movement/exercise chart & please check out our other offerings @ www.sitacise.com & for contact information email us @ mbrown1@neo.rr.com


Your friends,

Kathy & Mark Brown, I.